Me? Dialysis…?
NO WAY.
NO not ME!

Me? Dialysis...?
NO WAY.
NO not ME!

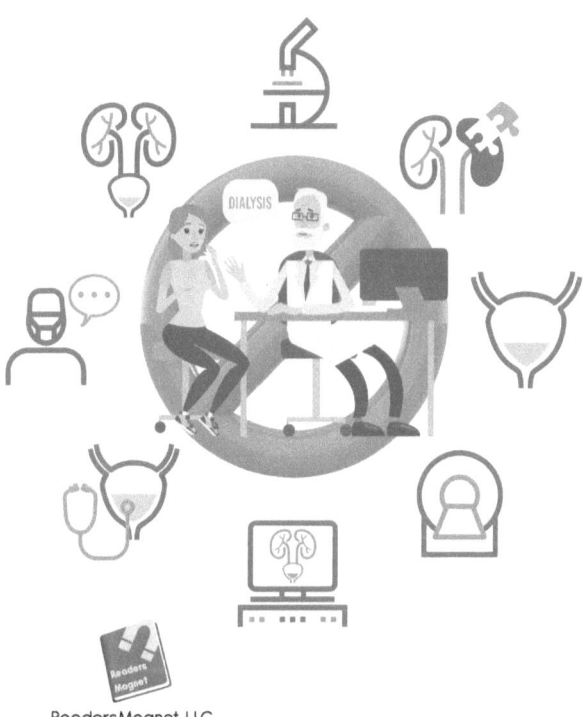

ReadersMagnet, LLC

Jolande Wijks

Me? Dialysis…? NO WAY. NO not ME!
Copyright © 2020 by Jolande Wijks

Published in the United States of America
ISBN Paperback: 978-1-950947-96-6
ISBN eBook: 978-1-950947-97-3

All rights reserved. No part of this publication may be reproduced, stored in a retrieval system or transmitted in any way by any means, electronic, mechanical, photocopy, recording or otherwise without the prior permission of the author except as provided by USA copyright law.

The opinions expressed by the author are not necessarily those of ReadersMagnet, LLC.

ReadersMagnet, LLC
10620 Treena Street, Suite 230 | San Diego, California, 92131 USA
1.619.354.2643 | www.readersmagnet.com

Book design copyright © 2020 by ReadersMagnet, LLC. All rights reserved.
Cover design by Ericka Walker
Interior design by Shemaryl Evans

I express my special words of gratitude to Mrs. Anita Fawcett (Canada) who made the translation into English of a great part of this book, in a very short time available. You were there at the right time and on the right place to help me realize this project and thus contributed in creating more awareness about dialysis in other Communities. Thank you so much, Anita.

Contents

1: I Hate My Mother! 9
2: I feel good, right? I'm perfectly healthy! 11
3: Bella thought peeing was disgusting 14
4: If only I was wearing my seatbelt 17
5: Gertrude has lots of pain 20
6: If only I had known it… 24
7: I really want to do an MRI 26
8: My baby doll won't lack anything! 28
9: Jenny is pregnant 31
10: Courage with Whiskey 33
11: Jessica knows better 38
12: Chandra 45

Glossary 50

With approval and thanks to Dr. Ken Berend, an Internist attached to the St. Elisabeth Hospital as Coordinating Medical Head of the Internal Department and the Curacao Dialysis Center; both located in Curacao.

My thanks also go to Nurse Gloria Mathew, former head nurse of the Dialysis Department of the St Elisabeth Hospital in Curacao, and Ms. Mariella Fernando, chairman of the Kidney Foundation Curacao, the former Netherlands Antilles.

1

I Hate My Mother!

Only after the midwife gave Erwin a slap on his buttocks, did he begin crying. It soon became clear that Erwin barely had any wet diapers after his birth. Following the doctor's examination of the baby, he told the new mother there was a congenital kidney abnormality. She should ensure Erwin always remained under strict control of the pediatrician because this disease could easily be controlled with medication. Erlisa, who was barely seventeen years old, had not even finished her schooling because of the teenage pregnancy, lack of money and her social conditions. She didn't understand half of what the doctor explained to her about her baby. She came from a very poor family. Her boyfriend, Isaac, who was almost as young as she was, did not even realize he had become a father and what that meant. When Erwin was a month old, she brought him to Isaac and his parents, left him there and disappeared. Erwin grew up with his father and his grandparents.
Erlisa had abandoned her baby of a few weeks because she couldn't handle the situation. Isaac was only an eighteen year old teenager without a sense of responsibility. He was also still

in school. Never again did Erlisa look back at her baby. She had also kept a deep secret about Erwin regularly requiring doctor checkups due to his malfunctioning kidneys. No one, not even his father, was aware of this. Only when Erwin was 20, after he became seriously ill and was admitted to the Intensive Care Unit to immediately begin dialysis, did his mother come out of nowhere and tell her story. The evil was unfortunately already irreversible; Erwin had never received the necessary treatment and medication, so he had to start dialysis in his twentieth year.

Erwin, now 27 years old, has been on dialysis for seven years. He hates his mother from the bottom of his heart. "Thanks to my mother, I now need dialysis to stay alive. I hate her. I don't consider her to be my mother. My grandma and grandpa are my parents. They have taken good care of me," stated Erwin, who wipes away a tear while telling funny stories about his grandparents and father.

2

I feel good, right? I'm perfectly healthy!

Kurti is 39 years old.
He feels good and says that he is perfectly healthy.
"I swim once a week to stay in shape. Every Saturday I work out for two hours in the gym; don't you see how muscular I am?" he asks his colleagues with a raised chest. They happen to remind him of his dodged annual checkups.
"But Kurt, you and I started military service together, we have been working together for ten years and always you dodge the annual medical checkup. Why?"
"Syslin, will you leave me alone? I feel good, eat well, and perform well. With three women and six children I have enough evidence. Do you want to be my fourth wife? Then you have to bear two children for me." he jokes.

"Seriously Kurti, you complain about headaches sometimes? Do you know why you get headaches?"

"Sysje, stop wearing me down! Save your energy for your husband and children. This is the ninth time you make my head weary with this subject. Don't let there be a tenth time; I'm warning you. I'm perfectly healthy. Listen, this is just a rumor and don't tell umm… Rudi, Ria's husband, has recently been to the doctor because he wasn't feeling well. He got a tablet that he had to take every night!"

"And… what was his problem?" Syslyn asked, not very impressed.

"Did you know that he couldn't properly use his, "tool" anymore?"

"Why? What do you mean?"

"He became impotent, Sysje…"

"Do you know what was wrong, what kind of a tablet it was or did he have a problem?"

"I don't know and I don't wanna know. Don't worry. Do you think I would waste my time going to a laboratory and sitting there for hours to be tortured by an ugly laboratory assistant armed with a thick needle? I would have to go to the doctor for results and perhaps even get prescribed medicine and after that, I might not be able to use my, "blunt needle" anymore? No, no, no. I'm fine. I'm vital and strong. I've got lots to do. My women like me the way I am and I don't want to experience what happened to Rudi. Absolutely and certainly not! Maybe I can give you two kids?" he added laughing. Syslyn shook her head and let the conversation go for what it was.

With sadness, Kurt often thinks of this past conversation with his colleague. Today is exactly one year since he was urgently admitted to the Intensive Care Unit with chronic kidney failure based on prolonged untreated hypertension. He never expected this; his world has a totally different color now. His arrogance has dropped to zero. Still, he cannot believe he almost died. Urgent dialysis saved him. His kidneys were so damaged by untreated hypertension that he escalated from an acute to a chronic dialysis patient.

If only I had listened to Syslin 12 years ago, he wrote on a note for the dialysis nurse who always welcomed him with a broad smile. The sister took the note, read it and looked at him without comprehending.

3

Bella thought peeing was disgusting

Bella was a thirteen year old girl that
looked like any normal teenager.
However, she had a phobia: she wouldn't use any other
toilet than the one in her own home. Some people made
jokes about it but not many paid too much attention to it.
Bella never urinated in school, when visiting relatives or
when she was in a restaurant or any other public place. What
Bella's parents didn't know was that Bella secretly threw
out the drinks she brought to school and drank as little
as possible; just to prevent having to go to the toilet. She
thought all toilets were disgusting and eventually she even
thought that about urinating. She didn't want to pee and
often held her urine for very long periods.
Her parents didn't have a clue about any medical problems.
Her mother did do the best to keep their toilet extra clean for
her daughter. She was proud of her daughter and told anyone
who would listen how "tidy" her Bella was. She also did her
best in school.
One day Bella came home from school and, as always,
she went straight to the toilet. But that day she stayed on

the toilet for hours. When her mother noticed this, she knocked on the door of the bathroom and asked, "Bella why are you in there so long?" It remained silent. Her mother went inside.

"Mom… I can't pee!" Bella cried.

"What's wrong Bella? Why are you crying?" her shocked mother shrieked when she saw Bella crying as she sat convulsing on the toilet.

"I can't… pee!" Bella screamed. "Pain momma… pain…" she moaned while squirming herself in all directions on the toilet. Immediately, the panicked mother wrapped a sheet around her daughter and brought her to the family doctor. The doctor determined her bladder was full and urgently referred them to the urologist. It appeared she had suffered a hefty urinary tract infection with her urine so concentrated and thickened, her ureter was clogged. The urologist had to catheterize her to extract the urine. And, as if that wasn't enough, he also found kidney stones in her renal pelvis which had significantly affected the functioning of her kidneys. Because Bella drank so little and had a proclivity for kidney stones, huge kidney stones had formed in her renal pelvis which had severely damaged the kidneys.

In the meantime, the internist was called to co-treat Bella; he really wanted a talk with the mother and daughter. "Where do I start…" he said hesitantly as he looked from Bella to her mother and back. After a deep sigh, he began, "Ma'am your daughter is still very young and still attends school. Currently, her problem of not being able to urinate was solved by the urologist and he has already told you this. Unfortunately, she's got more problems. The presence of kidney stones in your daughter's renal pelvis has caused "havoc" in her kidneys. Both kidneys are damaged but the right one much more than the left one."

The mother was petrified as she listened to the internist. She felt weird and dizzy… Like in a dream she heard the words, "Your daughter must be on dialysis.

"No… No…" she screamed as she held her head tight and kept shaking it back and forth. Bella quietly cried along with her mother. At that time she didn't really understand what awaited her and why. It did catch her attention that she had to go on dialysis soon to save her life. She wondered, what was dialysis?

4

If only I was wearing my seatbelt

It was a sunny day; a good day for the family to hit the road. However, Chapo had other plans. He longed to go for a fast ride in his new sports car all by himself. A week ago he had bought a 1992 Camaro. For years he had longed for such a car. Finally, at the age of thirty, after lots of hard work and sacrifice, he succeeded. It was his dream car. He treated it as a brand new car and polished it every day. Chapo loved speeding but couldn't get what he wanted within the city limits.

Despite the pleas of his wife and children, this time he didn't take them with him. He wanted to go racing!

"How can I race with my wife and children?" he thought.

Chapo got into his car and drove towards Banda Bou (the western part of Curaçao). Since he had quite a belly and was a bit heavier, he leaned back into the driver's seat, pushing his seat to the furthest setting. He felt like a king! No chattering kids voices in the back seat, no wife who would complain to him about her work, the rising prices in the grocery store, that his clothes were too tight for his big belly, diets where people lose weight and especially, nobody who told him to wear his seatbelt. He thought that was the worst and had already been caught three times at traffic checks; he still hadn't paid any of the fines.

It felt awesome to speed in his Camaro with the seat fully reclined. He kept increasing the speed feeling the rush of excitement. 120 kilometers per hour, not bad, he thought aloud as he approached a sharp curve without reducing speed. Then it happened… Bham… bradabap, boom… Camaro… Chapo and all, flipped over.

The accident happened so very fast. He had heard a loud noise and felt as if he'd fallen into a spinning washing machine before he violently smashed into something solid. Eyewitnesses reported Chapo being catapulted from the vehicle. Local residents found him unconscious and meters away from his precious car, right beside a tree. The paramedics of the ambulance service rushed him to the emergency room. When he woke up after many hours, he said he had suddenly seen a big black donkey in the middle of the road just beyond the curve.

He only recalled that he had hit the brakes hard but couldn't remember much more. After treatment, he was admitted with several fractures and a large contusion in his right kidney. His right kidney was severely damaged. He lay there with a lot of pain and had to have several scans and MRI's done.

Silent with grief, his worried wife and children were waiting for the doctor to come and talk with them. Eventually, a doctor with a flapping white coat and serious expression on his face approached them. "Mr. Chapo, what actually happened to you?" he asked after the introductions.

Weakly, Chapo told his whole story again.

"Were you wearing your seatbelt, sir?"

"No, doctor," he quietly said with much regret. He couldn't look his wife in the eyes, he felt that guilty.

"Mr. Chapo, did you know that you could have been dead right now and that you only have one kidney?"

"Absolutely not, doctor. It never bothered me. What do you mean… one kidney?" Startled and full of questions, Chapo looked at the doctor but didn't have the energy to speak further.

"I'm sorry, Mr. Chapo, you must understand that we have thoroughly examined and scanned your whole body because of the multiple injuries you sustained. We have detected that you only have one kidney in your body's right half and it seems that kidney is irreparably damaged by the car accident. You were probably born with only one kidney and you never knew. You have to start dialysis. From now on you'll be living without kidneys…"

5

Gertrude has lots of pain

Gertrude is 65 years old and has had almost no health concerns. She walks with her girlfriend, Trinaliena, five times a week and swims three times a week with Bertha, her twin sister. All three ladies feel full of vitality and were enjoying their well-deserved retirement after working together in banking for years. Bertha was the first to notice that there was something wrong with Gertrude.

"Gertrude, you can't keep up to me with swimming anymore, what's wrong? If I have done ten lengths you have only done six. Is something wrong with you? Are you not feeling well or are you in love?" Bertha asked with a smile.

"You know I don't like to complain; I'm usually a happy person, but lately the pain in my joints has been bothering me a lot. I've been feeling like this for a few weeks and it's gotten worse; even painkillers haven't helped a bit. Sometimes the pain makes me want to scream, but I refrain from doing that. This is why I called Trinaliena twice last week to cancel our walks. I was in too much pain. Do you think it's my age?" Gertrude asked seriously.

"Hmm… what does the doctor say?" inquired Bertha.

"Doctor? You know I don't deal with doctors, remember? They will never become rich because of me, you know." Gertrude stammered.

"Well, seriously now, if you're sick you should go see your family doctor, don't you think? Shall I make an appointment for you?" Bertha generously offered.

"Knowing you, I'm sure you would keep nagging me so go ahead."

During a short visit to her family doctor, Gertrude was told that she probably had gout but to confirm the diagnosis, she was referred to the laboratory to give some blood samples. Trinaliena joined her to the lab appointment. A week later, Gertrude had to see her family doctor to get the results. Of course, Bertha went with her because she really felt for her twin sister. It was like she felt what Gertrude felt. She knew when her sister was in pain, she didn't talk much and she had hardly said a word. So, someone had to go with her, besides she loved Gertrude.

"Good morning ladies. I have the results for you, Ms. Gertrude. The results are what I expected. Your uric acid level in your blood is very high. I have an excellent medicine for you." he said as he wrote a prescription.

"But doctor, how did you get a diagnosis this quickly? Are you sure it's gout? Shouldn't she go to the internist?" inquired Trinaliena.

"Oh no, she doesn't have to go to the internist," answered the doctor, "she'll have to take just one tablet twice a day to feel relief very soon. It's an approved medicine; don't you worry. Come back and see me in two weeks for a checkup."

Bertha wanted to ask more questions but Gertrude had already gotten up and was walking towards the door. She was in so much pain; she wanted to pick up the approved medicine at the pharmacy as soon as possible. She went straight home clutching her prescription. After taking her first dose of the medication, she decided to go to bed because the pain was so unbearable. When she woke up after a short restless sleep, she felt strange. She couldn't describe the feeling, but attributed it to fatigue and stress. She never wanted to go to the doctor and hated the long wait at the pharmacy to get her medication. She was quite annoyed at the pharmacy assistant who couldn't understand that she had to hurry. The pain made her feel very agitated.

As evening set in, Gertrude took her second tablet and went to bed early.

The next morning her body felt hot and she woke up very ill. She couldn't get up!

Startled, she picked up the phone and called Bertha to come see her. Bertha called Trinaliena and together they went to visit Gertrude. She had been a childless widow for five years and lived alone. She almost never complained so when she did, it had to be serious. Gertrude stayed in bed; she felt lousy but was glad that her sister and girlfriend had a key to her house. She had never felt so sick and weak and didn't even have the strength to turn around in bed.

"What the hell happened to me? Am I dead?" she mumbled. When the women arrived they were completely shocked to see Gertrude so sick. "What's that rash on your body? What did you eat?" they inquired.

Only when asked, had Gertrude looked down at her own body seeing a strange rash on her extremities; large and small red pimples. Not wasting any time, they helped Gertrude to the emergency room. After obtaining her medical history, the internist performed various blood examinations, x-rays and scans. It was ascertained that she had sustained interstitial nephritis by taking Allopurinol, the anti-gout medication that she had taken with confidence because her family doctor had prescribed it for her. To make matters worse she was told that her only salvation was acute dialysis. Her first reaction: "No… Me… Dialysis… No Way!"

6

If only I had known it...

It was a rainy day. Ronny had a habit of grabbing a beer at the Snack (a typical small bar/restaurant found in the Caribbean) after work. He wasn't a real drinker but enjoyed being a social drinker. It had become a habit that his wife and children weren't really happy with because sometimes he came home very late and grumpy. The rain that day didn't stop him from meeting his friends at the Snack. His friends were less noisy today and acted a bit mysterious. "What were they doing on the street with that strange car in the rain?" Ronny wondered aloud. Right afterwards, he asked himself this again, as his friends gathered around him. Just as suddenly as the strange car had appeared, it disappeared.
"What were you guys up to just now?" Ronny asked.
"We have a surprise for you! Next week is your birthday and we've already found something nice for you."
"And what would that be?" Ronny asked curiously.
"The rain has stopped now so come with us," teased the group.
Curious and happy that his friends had an early birthday surprise for him, he followed. They went to a secluded table

that was behind a tree and out of sight of the other Snack visitors. The five friends formed a circle around the table. Solemnly, Brian pulled out five small packages. "To your birthday and long live our friendships! First, Ronny then Rene, Jason, Dirk and this one is mine" Brian said as he distributed the packages.

Ronny felt the hairs on the back of his neck go up. It was an illegal substance! He took the package in his hand and recognized the white powder. He had seen it in movies often enough but this was the first time in real life. He had never been in favor of any drugs whatsoever but didn't want to disappoint his friends. They had arranged this for him and had all participated…

So Ronny began a new habit which didn't stop after one try. Exactly nine months after this life changing birthday present, he felt so sick he ended up in the emergency room. He suffered from a persistent chest pain, palpitations, terrible sweating, was short of breath and obviously very anxious. The usual examinations showed he had suffered acute renal failure due to cocaine intoxication; Ronny now needed acute dialysis or he wouldn't survive.

He had regret, regret and more regret when this bad news sunk in. If he had known this in advance, he would have never participated in that cocaine trend; the worst birthday present ever!

7

I really want to do an MRI

Margreta Slinger, a forty-eight-year-old woman has been complaining for weeks about a sore left side and back. Her family doctor has prescribed several painkillers with moderate success. On her third visit to the doctor with the same symptoms, he decided to take an x-ray of her back and her left side. There was nothing worth mentioning to be seen on the x-ray.

"Again, nothing noticeable, doc? I'm tired of these pains. Urine is good, my blood results are fine; what the hell is going on? Could you please book me for an MRI scan? I would like to know what this is. Could it be cancer? Almost every day I hear of someone dying of cancer. I really want to undergo the MRI, doc."

"Too many X-rays aren't good for your body and furthermore…" replied the Doctor.

"Stop doc… it's my body. I want to do the MRI!" she said impatiently. She didn't even let the doctor finish or allow any interference; no more excuses. Sighing, the disgruntled doctor gave her the application; the MRI was booked the same day.

Margreta was apprehensive of the examination but knew it would eventually end, so she persevered. While she was getting dressed afterwards and looking forward to going home, she suddenly felt a strange sensation in her body. It seemed as if her body was on fire; she began to scream. The laboratory technician rushed to her and asked her what was going on. She grabbed his arms and begged him for help. Her body was burning with fever. She felt excruciating pain and thought she was going to die. The laboratory technician saw Margreta was shaking throughout her entire body and he wondered if she was having an epileptic seizure.

She kept a convulsive hold on the laboratory technician's arm and together they fell to the floor. With great difficulty, the laboratory technician freed himself and alerted his colleagues. Several employees, including the radiologist, came running. Immediately, the radiologist injected some medication into her. Margreta had suffered a severe allergic reaction to the radio contrast agent that she had been injected intravenously in order to undergo the MRI. The allergy was so severe that she urgently was admitted into the Intensive Care Unit. The radio contrast agent had caused extensive damage to her organs and had paralyzed her kidneys. The insistence of Margreta to undergo the MRI came at a very high price; she needed acute dialysis due to the sudden loss of function of both her kidneys, as a result of this allergic reaction.

8

My baby doll won't lack anything!

Perla didn't go to school today; she just didn't feel like it... again. Flora, her mother, was fed up with begging her daughter to go to school and retreated to her luxurious room to let her tears of frustration run freely. Being a fifty-year-old widow with only one precious ten year old child, she felt her daughter was the only thing left from her late husband, Rodney. He worked hard and with lots of prayers and the considerable inheritance he left her after being killed in the Middle Eastern war, she was trying hard to raise her daughter right.
It had been five years since her beloved Rodney's tragic death and she wasn't getting used to parenting on her own. She enjoyed not having to work and having almost everything she desired, but with sadness she thinks of him. Her only feeling of happiness was thinking about her most precious pearl; her daughter, Perla. She was such a beautiful child and there was only one thing she would physically change about her; Perla had been a diabetic since she was eight years old. Being insulin dependent, you would think she would understand the importance of the lifestyle required by diabetics but she rebelled more and more as she got older.

She didn't want to stick to her diet or her insulin routine. She only injected insulin when she deemed it absolutely necessary, sometimes leaving it way too long. Despite loving Perla more than anything, Flora felt that her daughter could choose to do what she wanted, as long as she was happy.

"Mommy…" Perla screamed from her playroom. Flora rushed to her daughter. "You want to go to school today, don't you?" she asked her daughter with a pleading voice.

"I told you that I don't want to go to school today, remember? Come play with me mommy. I want to play nurse and doctor. Today all my dolls get a shot."

"Did you inject yourself, Sweety?"

"No, no and today I won't! I want to drink a cola and have a cheesecake for breakfast my sweet mommy."

"Sure, Sweety." Flora answered.

Flora perfectly knew what her daughter was and wasn't allowed to have as a diabetic. On the other hand, she didn't want her daughter to be sad, so she made sure her daughter wouldn't be lacking anything. Her baby doll always got her way and her mom consciously missed checkup visits to the doctor on purpose. This uncontrolled diabetes and high glucose diet led to irreversible organ damage, particularly renal failure.

Perla got sick… sick as a dog. Flora felt terrible and begged the doctors and nurses to help her daughter. She even offered extra money so her daughter would be well taken care of. From the moment she was in hospital, she didn't leave her side. Perla was put on a very strict diet and her medication and insulin was strictly implemented by the nursing staff. Flora had finally come to realize that she should have never given her daughter a free reign. She had raised her totally wrong. She regretted it like no other and felt like she had disappointed her beloved Rodney.

There was another setback for Flora when she was told that Perla also needed dialysis. She could no longer handle the situation and had immense feelings of guilt about the severity of the illness of her most precious pearl. To make matters worse, not even a year after starting dialysis, Perla suddenly died due to severe heart failure. Her vital organs were so severely affected by her mother allowing poor eating habits (especially her uncontrolled craving for sweets) and allowing Perla to skip her insulin injections. A mother who wanted everything for her child just gave too much of the wrong things…

9

Jenny is pregnant

Jenny got pregnant for the very first time
when she was 35 years old.
She felt so fortunate yet, despite that she dreaded doctor's
appointments. She promised herself not to miss any
appointments for the health of her unborn baby. She
wanted to have a perfect pregnancy and a healthy baby.
At one of her appointments, he told her that her blood
pressure was slightly elevated. She was advised to
consume less sodium and be mindful of her diet. She
was very strict with her diet and delivered a healthy
baby without any incidents during her pregnancy.
She managed her blood pressure well throughout the
pregnancy, but her doctor advised her not to have more
children because of the high blood pressure that could
be a conflict in future pregnancies. High blood pressure
has afflicted the health of her family for generations.
After five years, Jenny got pregnant with her second child.
This time she was hospitalized with a dangerously high
blood pressure. It went up to 220/130. She was restricted
to bedrest. After one month in the hospital her blood

pressure was still dangerously high. She wasn't feeling good
at all. She was nauseated, vomiting, had no appetite and
was sleeping almost all the time. They moved her to a dark
room but she was still feeling like everything was rolling in
her head, just like she was in a big roller coaster that never
seemed to end. Jenny remembered that she got a morphine
shot from the nurse and after that she was gone…
The next day the doctor woke her up, explained her situation
and told her that she had to have urgent surgery to save herself
and her baby's life. In a sleepy voice she asked the doctor:
'Please do surgery for me to never have any children anymore.'
After about seven days, she woke up in the Intensive
Care Unit with her family beside her bed. She learned
that she gave birth to a baby boy who was in the
incubator. After the section caesarian they urged her to
the ICU because of her grave situation. She developed
Rhabdomyolyses. Her family could hardly recognize her.
She had Anasarca; swollen all over her body, she couldn't
see, couldn't urinate. Her kidneys and liver were down.
That's were Jenny got dialysis treatments. According to her
doctor she was suffering from acute kidney failure because of
eclampsia. She had to start acute hemodialysis to save her life.
After two months she stopped her dialysis treatments,
because her kidneys function returned to normal.
For two years she lived with a constant need for medication,
but no dialysis. But then her kidney function started to
deteriorate to the point that she had to start with dialysis all
over again. This time she had the opportunity to get ahead of
her disease so she choose to start with peritoneal dialysis.
Jenny was already aware that the world of dialysis was
not easy, but she was grateful to have the treatment
option that would help her be there for her children.

10

Courage with Whiskey.

Armand, was a well-known actor for five years. The leader of
his theater group; Sherwin, was married to Ana, a lady from the
Dominican Republic who was running a bar nearby Armand's
home. On his way to work Armand always passes the bar.
Most of the time it was busy, especially in the evenings. Loud
conversations and laughter could be heard from a distance.
Armand waved and drove quickly to his home. He was not
used to visiting the bar but his colleagues did on a daily basis.
His parents had passed away years ago but he could
still hear his mother's voice: "Armand never become a
regular bar visitor. The ladies will take your money. You
will give into them. Your life will become a hell etc."
His parents raised him as a catholic and as their only child,
he wanted to make them proud. Until his thirtieth birthday.
His colleagues set up a surprise party for him. They brought
him a life-sized gift in a wheelbarrow. Armand was very
happy. He never really had a birthday party. Sometimes
he even forgot his own birthday. He was curious about
his gift. "That big? Was it a refrigerator maybe?"
His colleagues brought him snacks and a lot of alcoholic drinks.

In daily life Armand was very shy, but at work he was different. On stage he could do anything. That was his life. Stage fright was not in his dictionary. However in daily life he had no courage to look for a girlfriend. His colleagues were aware of that, that's why they made a plan. Armand had no idea.
The party was all fun; eating, drinking, telling stories, laughing, until midnight. Time to open his present. He had to climb a stepping stool to cut the big red ribbon on top of the Big Box. He noticed that there were some holes on the box. Peeping through the holes he saw something as red as the ribbon. Suddenly he felt strange, almost afraid of the Big Box.
Just as he was about to cut the ribbon, someone shouted: "Stop" It was Sherwin. "Carla can you help me blindfold Armand" Everyone started singing and clapping.
Carla was one of his colleagues who spoke a lot with Armand. It didn't bother her that he was not much of a speaker. Most of the time she would intentionally involve him in her conversations. Armand liked her a lot but never showed it. He was always very polite and correct with women, almost afraid of them. Maybe his mom had told him too many rules on how to handle women.
Carla blindfolded Armand and helped guide him through the cutting process.
Under loud whistling, clapping and screaming, Carla pulled the cloth from his eyes. He looked and got the shock of his life. He couldn't believe his eyes. He was blinking and rubbing his eyes with his hands. Standing there with his mouth wide open, he couldn't say anything. He was perplexed.
Carla saw that his face changed colors and that he was wobbling. She grabbed him and helped keep him on his feet.
"Only for you and you alone" Sherwin shouted half drunk.

"Isn't she beautiful" said Carla, while pointing to his
present, a young lady in a red dress, who was smiling
and looking at Armand with a provocative look.
Someone offered him a drink and happy that he could
do something he grabbed the glass and drunk the
content with a gulp. He felt his throat burning but had
no time to pay attention to that burning sensation.
Nikita the lady in the red dress, knew what she wanted. She
climbed with grace out of the Big Box, walked towards Armand
and gave him a tender kiss on his mouth. Armand didn't know
what was happening. His face turned red, almost purple. He
asked for a drink and got the same thing he got before. He
felt better after this second glass and was getting loose.
He understood that Nikita was twenty five years old and
was the niece of Ana, Sherwin's wife. She was also from
the Dominican Republic and was longing to marry a man
from the Caribbean. Ana thought that Armand would be a
good husband for her. That's why they wrapped her as a big
present for Armand. Armand was the only bachelor in the
company. All of them, especially Nikita liked that plan.
Meanwhile Armand noticed that he had the courage to
approach Nikita. The more whiskey he had, the more courage.
The next day Armand woke up with a heavy head. To his
horror he noticed that he wasn't alone. Slowly but certainly
he remembered what had happened the night before. He
could hardly believe that he got a human present and that
he slept with her. How was this possible? He felt very guilty
and was thinking about his mother and her words. He
then quickly took a shower and went to visit Sherwin.
Ignoring the invitation of Sherwin to go inside, he stayed at
the door to talk with him. He told Sherwin that he couldn't
accept the present because he was feeling bad and guilty.

Sherwin listened to Armand, stared at him for a minute, went inside, came back, and handed him a big paper bag with contents. He said: Go home and pour yourself a glass and enjoy your present. Life is too short to worry. Act like you're on a stage my son."
Armand went home. The first thing he did when he arrived home was peep into his bedroom. Nikita was sleeping in his bed as if she never slept anywhere else. Armand went in the kitchen and inspected the paper bag. A big bottle of Jack Daniels. He did what Sherwin told him to do. He drank a full glass in one go and felt more confident already. Now he could handle Nikita. He could handle anything. He was not feeling drunk, but just a little tipsy. Any nervousness, uncertainty or shyness disappeared after drinking whiskey. A new era was starting for him. He started drinking whiskey on a daily basis. The number of glasses was increasing day by day. Armand became addicted. Nobody was bothered. On the contrary, Armand was participating in everything. He was loose. He also visited the bar regularly. Nikita was helping her aunt regularly at the bar. Every time Armand visited she poured him whiskey because that was all he drank. Despite his alcohol abuse, he behaved all the time. With whiskey in his system he was talkative, indulgent and very charming towards Nikita. What he didn't realize, was that slowly but surely this whiskey habit was causing irreparable damage to his body. Almost every morning when he went to the bathroom, he was thinking about his mother's words. At those moments he felt so ashamed and dirty that he took a shower to feel clean again. Then he went to work and after work he would hurry to enjoy himself with Nikita and his favorite drink at the bar. That's how his life was going day after day, month after month until he started complaining of stomach pains. He

made an appointment with his primary care physician and got
medication for his stomach. He didn't tell the doctor anything
about his drinking habit and went on drinking on a daily basis.
Just two years after the doctor's visit, Armand collapses on
the stage. He was having pain in the flanks for a while. He
was also experiencing foamy urine, nausea and vomiting but
was ignoring it. Instead he was 'drinking his pain away'.
He was rushed to the hospital in an Ambulance. After different
blood tests, urine tests, X-rays and other diagnostic tests, the
results showed a big stomach ulcer, a malfunctioning liver and a
damaged kidney with very low kidney function. All because of
his favorite drink. His kidneys were only functioning at 10%.
His life changed completely. He couldn't act anymore
because of the lack of energy. His kidney failure was the
reason that he had a low red cell count, causing him to be
weak and lacking energy. He couldn't not work anymore.
Armand had no income. Nikita vanished without a
trace. His colleagues hardly had time for him.
He stayed alone and realized more than ever that he should
never have started drinking alcohol, not for courage, not for
any reason. It has caused only misery. He was confronted
with something he had never expected or even thought about:
Dialysis! He didn't even know the meaning of Dialysis.
With endless pain, from one day to the next he
was introduced to the world of dialysis.
Slowly but surely he realized what he had done
to himself. He had literally drank his health and
peaceful social life to pieces with whiskey.

11

Jessica knows better

Jessica was bored one day, and she was looking
through an old magazine. She hated to wait.
She didn't want to come to this place.
"What am I doing here" was she asking herself. She knew, but
she didn't want to remind herself. If it wasn't for Robby, she
would not be here. She was annoyed with the other people in
the waiting room. They sat calmly as if they had all the time
in the world. Most of them were just sitting, staring around,
while some of them were reading a newspaper or a book.
Nobody was complaining. Robby was one of them he looked
like a Zombie. Every now and then he'd lay his hands on her
knee, to reassure her or... did he do that because he wanted
to make sure that Jessica was still sitting on that chair?
For days Jessica was complaining of a burning sensation
while urinating but didn't want to go to the doctor. Robby
her fiancée was begging her to get to the doctor, but she
refused. Despite that Jessica had a very stubborn personality,
she didn't like to go to the doctor and hated to take
medications. She remembered that when she was a little
girl, she was always vomiting when her mom forced her to
take medications. She was getting nauseous and threw up.

Only when Jessica felt a heavy pain under her belly and
her urine was so smelly that Robby had to comment about
it, despite her reluctance she decided to listen to Robby.
Robby and Jessica stood up together when
the doctor called her name.
"No Robby, I'll go alone. Wait for me" she said.
Robby didn't like that, but sat down again. He would have
liked to accompany her but didn't want to create a scene.
He was so curious what she would tell the doctor and what
the doctor would decide, but sat down quietly. He could feel
the eyes of the people in the room staring right at him.
After five minutes Jessica came out angry.
"Let's go" she said.
Robby waved to the doctor who was standing at the door of
his office and nodded to the people in the waiting room. The
doctor shook his head while watching them leave the room.
Robby drove the car with Jessica next to him, home
without speaking to each other. He was looking at
her through the corners of his eyes. She was leaning
backwards in her seat with her eyes closed. He didn't
want to ask anything now. She looked very unsatisfied.
Arrived at home, he couldn't hold on anymore.
"What did the doctor told you Jess?"
"I will tell you in a minute, I got to go to the bathroom"
When she came back, she told Robby that the doctor
told her that she had a urinary tract infection. He
wrote her a prescription and told her to drink a lot.
"I always tell you to drink a lot of
water…" Robby interrupted her.
"Don't start" she shouted. "I know how much I
have to drink and nobody decides for me."
Trying to change the subject he asked:
"What prescription did you get?"

"How should I know? It's in my purse.'
"But you need the medications though…"
"Robby, I'm in pain, can you leave me alone?"
"May I have the prescription, so I can go get the medications for you" he asked calmly while he handed her a glass of fresh orange juice.
Jessica gave him an angry look while reluctantly handing him the prescription. Robby ignored her look, took the prescription went to the pharmacy and came back with the medications. He gave it to Jessica. He was happy that she had drunk all her orange juice.
Robby knows that his partner was surly and stubborn most of the time, but he had a lot of patience with her because he loved her.
"Nitrofurantoin" Jessica was reading out loud. "4 times a day 1 caps of 100mg. Finish the treatment… hum… Tylenol extra strength 4 times a day 500 mg PRN for pain."
"Take them" he said.
"Yeah, I guess I have to." She said calmly.
Robby was happy with her answer and hoped that she really meant what she said.
The next day Robby noticed that Jessica was complaining less and was even laughing with him. The bad smell that she left behind after using the bathroom was also gone. Life went on.
Exactly two weeks later, she noticed when undressing that her panties had some blood on it. She was shocked. She was sure that she didn't have her period. It wasn't that time and she had a regular menstrual cycle. She was checking her panties and noticed a strange odor. It smelled like rotten eggs. Angrily she threw it in the garbage.
She thought about her doctor's visit two weeks ago. Her doctor was asking her personal questions, but when he noticed that

she wasn't interested and almost disrespectful, he cut of the
conversation and wrote the prescription. He also tried to give
her some advice but she didn't listened. The only thing she
remembered was that she had to drink a lot. She felt that
the doctor was annoyed because of her attitude but it didn't
bother her. That day, she was not in the mood for questions
and advise. She never liked interference in her private life.
She took a shower and went to bed. She didn't get much
sleep that night. The next day she got up and was in pain.
When she got up from the toilet to flush her urine, she was
shocked. The toilet bowl was red. There was only blood.
"My God, what's wrong with me, did I pee blood?"
She flushed before Robby would see the blood. She had to
flush a couple times to get the toilet bowl clean. Quietly
she went to her wardrobe, searching and searching until
she grabbed a box with antibiotics. She had hidden the rest
of the antibiotics in her wardrobe. She only took 4. Why
would she finish them all if she was feeling better? She
drank the fresh made orange juice that Robby offered her.
Usually she didn't like to drink but those days she had drunk
at least one liter per day while Robby was watching her.
"What should I do, tell Robby or not? If I tell him he will
force me to go to that annoying doctor again. No I don't want
that." She took a tablet and decided to keep drinking a lot.
This time she took 6. She took them every four hours instead,
and didn't see any blood anymore. That was better she thought.
When she had no pain and didn't see any blood anymore, she
hid the rest of the pills again. Jessica went to work as usual.
She was working as a cashier at a fast-food restaurant. It was
always very busy. When she had the need to use the restroom,
she had to wait for another cashier and that could take a
long time. Her boss didn't trust all the workers with the cash

register. Meanwhile it became a habit that she would hold
her urine for a long time. Sometimes she dripped urine in her
panties but it didn't bother her. She kept working as usual.
"It smells like urine in here" a colleague said. "Yes, I smell it
too." She answered like she had nothing to do with that smell.
Jessica had a habit of cleaning herself from back to front after
urinating. She found it easier because she could easily look
and smell the toilet paper. That's why she got angry when
the doctor was asking her about her bathroom manners.
She didn't want interference in her private manners.
Jessica was not hygienic. In the last three months she
got five urinary tract infections. She just did her own
thing then. Drink a lot of water and take two of her
antibiotic pills. Robby didn't know anything about that.
That morning Jessica got up to go to the bathroom. She was
urinating blood again. Meanwhile she had no antibiotics
anymore. She thought she would drink a lot, but then she felt
some pain in her sides and under her belly. The pain got worse
and worse. She stumbled to her bed and curled herself into a
fetus position. She couldn't hide this pain from Robby because
she was crying and screaming. The pain was unbearable. She
vomited, urinated her pants and kept on rolling in her bed.
In panic Robby called his doctor, who sent
the ambulance to pick up Jessica.
After several tests in the hospital and information
from Jessica, the doctor came to explain her situation.
This time Robby got Jessica's permission to stay.
"Miss Jessica, it looks like you have had several urinary tract
infections in a short period of time. These infections were
not treated like they should have been, so the bacteria got
the chance to multiply and do more harm to your system.
Did you know that you have polycystic Kidney Disease?"
"No, what is that?"

"That is a congenital kidney disease. The kidneys
are not normal, they form cysts that prevent
the kidney from functioning normally."
"How did I get it?"
"Maybe you have relatives that also have polycystic kidneys?"
"No I don't know. I don't worry about my family and they
don't have to worry about me" She answered angrily.
"Anyway… your kidneys are not functioning
as they are supposed to be and…"
"When can I go home" Jessica interrupted the doctor.
"I'm sorry Jessica, you have to stay in the hospital for a while
and you need to have dialysis. You can't go home now. Your life
is in danger. Your kidneys are functioning at minimal capacity."
"Dialysis? You mean I have to clean my
blood through a machine?"
"Yes, you will have to dialyze 3 times a week, so you will be
on the machine for 4 hours. This machine will help do some
of the work that your kidneys are supposed to do, like get rid
of waste products and excessive fluids out of your blood."
"No, no…I can't, my boss won't let me. I need my work.
I need my own money. I can't become dependent on
anyone." She turned her back to Robby and the doctor."
The doctor left the room shrugging while Robby caressed
and comforted Jessica. It was a shock for both of them. Jessica
refused to go for dialysis, until she felt so sick it made her life
unbearable. She was constantly vomiting, couldn't urinate, her
upper and lower extremities were very edematous (swollen
with fluid). She couldn't sleep and couldn't breathe. She
felt like she was drowning. At that moment Jessica started
begging for treatment. The doctor came to visit her and left
her with a choice, to die or Stat dialysis. She chose the latter.
Jessica started dialysis, felt better and became a social person.
She lost her job but with help from the kidney foundation

she got another job. They all cared about her: The other patients, the staff of the dialysis clinic and the people of the Kidney foundation. She saw them every other day and soon they became good friends. Jessica transformed into a responsible, social and assisting dialysis patient.

12

Chandra

Many people found her name too difficult to pronounce. Others would think that it was too long. To make it easier Chandrika-Jai-Persadiatie shortened her name to Chandra. Everyone called her Chandra. She was always happy and busy. She didn't like to and couldn't sit still. Even if she was tired, she would still look for something to do. Her mom was a very polite lady who happened to be a tailor. Sitting behind her sewing machine all day long, she was trying to earn some money to help raise her eight kids. Her dad was a doorman at an apartment complex. Most of the time he was working extra hours. Chandra was the eldest of the eight daughters in the family. She was like her mother's right hand and felt responsible for her seven sisters. Chandra was eighteen years old and finished high school as a straight A student. She was studying to become a lawyer. Her dream was to earn a lot of money as a successful lawyer to help support her family. Everything Chandra was doing, she wanted to excel. She was making sure that her sisters were ready to go to school, their hair were well comb, she was helping them with their homework, She was doing the laundry and kept the house clean. Her mom had nothing to worry about.

In the mornings she would go to the college, in the afternoon she was busy with her sisters, doing the household chores or studying in the library. She never went to sleep without studying. She would never rest. They needed her for everything, at home and college. Her fellow students were inviting her to study together and they wanted her to take part in all sorts of activities. Chandra would never say no, even if she was tired. She would always help someone else first then think about herself. It was the last Friday of May. Two more weeks for Chandra and her fellow students to finish a thesis for school. Meanwhile her sisters were also busy with tests and exams. She went back and forth. Helping her sisters with their schoolwork in the afternoon, clean the house and do the laundry. Hurry to the library in the evenings, help her fellow students and go home do her own work late at night. That night she stayed awake until three am to do work on her own thesis. She was behind however she helped others to be on schedule. After typing the last words on her laptop she fell in a deep sleep. She did not eat nor shower that night.
At five her alarm went off. This morning Chandra was not feeling as energetic as usual. She felt strange. Every morning she was happy to get up and help her sisters especially on Saturdays when her sisters were at home. She was doing the laundry and the household chores while she was talking to them, listening to what they experienced at school because she liked that and thought it was very important. Sometimes she played games with them in between her work.
This Saturday morning she had a difficult time getting up. Something was wrong with her. What, was her big question. When she was ready to brush her teeth, she realized that she couldn't open her mouth widely. Her cheeks were stiff and her throat was sore. Why was her throat sore she was

asking herself. She was scared. She couldn't become sick
at this moment. What would her sisters do without her
help? Her mom and dad were relying on her. Even her
fellow students couldn't miss her. She was never sick.
With a lot of effort she brushed her teeth and rinsed her
mouth. She noticed that her mouth was still smelly, so
she was looking for the mouthwash. She found an empty
bottle. Her sisters probably used it all. Her mom bought a
big bottle of mouthwash once a month. Despite her mom
asking them to use it economically they would still use it in
abundance and finish the bottle before the end of the month.
Chandra's body was aching, but she had no time to pay
attention to herself. Her appetite was down, but she was
thinking that it was because of the sore throat. Her sisters
were telling her stories about what happened at school,
so she was listening and laughing with them, forgetting
about feeling sick. No one noticed her pain, not even
her fellow students. She kept her feelings to herself.
After two weeks Chandra's sore throat became worse
and her mouth was full of white patches. She could
hardly open her mouth and developed a fever. She was
holding her hand in front of her mouth when she was
talking. A foul smell was coming out of her mouth.
One of her sisters noticed that and told their mom.
"What's going on, why are you holding your hand in
front of your mouth when you're talking? Why is your
mouth smelling that bad?" her mom asked her.
Her mom looked into her mouth and saw the white
patches that were all over her throat and her tongue.
She also noticed that Chandra had a fever.
"You need to see a doctor Chandra"
"No mom, please no, I have so much to do and I
need to help my fellow college students."

Her mom was not even listening to her.
She called her husband right away to bring their
daughter to the doctor. Chandra was hesitating but
her mom and dad insisted so she let them.
The doctor had seen Chandra and referred
her with urgency to the hospital.
She had to be admitted and had all sort of tests.
They started her right away on antibiotics and
a specialist came to see her the next day.
He found out that Chandra was experiencing this
sore throat for 2 weeks, the patches in her mouth, less
appetite, nausea and even stomach pain for days. She
refused to go to the doctor because she wanted to
help her family and her fellow college students.
The doctor explained to her that she had developed post
streptococcal glomerulonephritis. Because she didn't get any
treatment for the throat infection, which was a streptococcal
infection. The bacteria got the chance to damage the
kidneys. That caused her kidney functions to go down.
Chandra couldn't believe her ears.
"Is that bad?" she asked.
"That is not all", said the doctor.
"Your kidney functions are so low that you need urgent dialysis"
"Dialysis? I don't have time for that, I have to
help my family and my fellow students."
"No Chandra, this time you have to help yourself.
You have to stop being altruistic."
That night was endless for Chandra. Dialysis, infection,
altruistic, all those words were tumbling in her head. The doctor
was right. She was always so passionate helping others first,
forgetting about herself. Now she was in trouble because of
that. She needed dialysis, because of an untreated infection.
"I'm a mess" she whispered and cried herself asleep.

Would you like to know more about your health regarding your kidneys?

Visit your doctor before it is too late and ask for a checkup with explanations of your:

    Glucose
    Blood pressure
    Creatinine
    Albumin in the urine.

When necessary, dialysis or kidney transplantation is a good alternative for people with kidney failure. However, avoid unpleasant surprises and cherish your kidneys. They purify your blood! Without your kidneys, you cannot live and you will need a kidney transplant or dialysis for the rest of your life.

Glossary

In acute renal failure, renal function rapidly deteriorates. The kidneys aren't able to remove sufficient waste materials from your blood. Renal function can deteriorate in a period of a few hours, days or weeks. This is called acute kidney disease or acute renal failure. (www.umcutrecht.nl)

Chronic renal insufficiency is a slow (months to years) progressive decrease of the ability of the kidneys to filter waste products of the metabolism from the blood.
(www.merckmanual.nl)

Cocaine intoxication is intoxication due to cocaine use.
(www.transplantatiestichting.nl)

Acute Interstitial Nephritis: is characterized by a progressive renal failure that develops within a few days.
(JJE van Everdingen – 2010)

Gout is a painful inflammation caused by crystallized uric

acid in a joint. Uric acid dissolves easily in warm blood but
a too high concentration of this acid can precipitate as small
needle-shaped crystals. The crystallization of uric acid in a
joint often leads to rapidly emerging severe inflammatory
reaction with redness, swelling, lots of pain, heat and loss
of function. Patients sometimes suddenly wake up in pain
at night and can often barely walk. Besides in the toes, gout
may also occur in other places, for example in the ankles,
knees, fingers or in the ears. (nl.wikipedia.org/wiki/Gout)
MRI is an abbreviation for magnetic resonance imaging. MRI
technology uses magnetic resonance to create images. These
images can be made of various body parts, for example the
brains or the lungs. So there is no need to make incisions in
the body. This is important for this method. One MRI use is
the detection of cancer cells. The technique of MRI is based
on the characteristic of a particle in the core (nucleus) of
the hydrogen atom. Protons are sensitive to magnetic fields.
(www.natuurkunde.nl/articles)

Caesarian section, also known as C-section, or caesarian
delivery, is the use of surgery to deliver babies. A caesarian
section is often necessary when a vaginal delivery
would put the baby or mother at risk. (Wikipedia)

Rhabdomyolysis is a condition in which damaged skeletal
muscle breaks down rapidly. Symptoms may include muscle
pains, weakness, vomiting and confusion. There may be tea-
colored urine or an irregular heartbeat. Some of the muscle
breakdown products, such as the protein myoglobin, are harmful
to the kidneys and may lead to kidney failure. (Wikipedia)

Anasarca is a severe and generalized form of edema, with
subcutaneous swelling throughout the body. (Wikipedia)

Eclampsia is a condition in which one or more convulsions occur in a pregnant woman suffering from high blood pressure, often followed by coma and posing a threat to the health of mother and baby. (Wikipedia)

Peritoneal Dialysis (PD) is a type of dialysis which uses the peritoneum in a person's abdomen as the membrane through which fluid and dissolved substances are exchanged with the blood. It is used to remove excess fluid, correct electrolyte problems, and remove toxins in those with kidney failure. Peritoneal dialysis has better outcomes than hemodialysis during the first couple of years. Other benefits include greater flexibility and better tolerability in those with significant heart disease. (Wikipedia)
Hemodialysis, also spelled haemodialysis or simply dialysis, is a process of purifying the blood of a person whose kidneys are not working normally. This type of dialysis achieves the extracorporeal removal of waste products such as creatinine and urea and free water from the blood when the kidneys are in a state of kidney failure. Hemodialysis is one of three renal replacement therapies (the other two being kidney transplant and peritoneal dialysis). (Wikipedia)

Polycystic kidney disease (PKD or PCKD, also known as polycystic kidney syndrome) is a genetic disorder in which the renal tubules become structurally abnormal, resulting in the development and growth of multiple cysts within the kidney. These cysts may begin to develop in utero, in infancy, in childhood, or in adulthood. Cysts are non-functioning tubules filled with fluid pumped into them, which ranged in size from microscopic to enormous, crushing adjacent normal tubules and eventually rendering them non-functional as well. (Wikipedia)

Post-Streptococcal Glomerulonephritis or PSGN is a rare kidney Disease that can develop after group A strep infections. (https://www.cdc.gov diseases public)